I0435413

Controlling blood sugar and curing diabetes

Manage your diabetes today with various
methods, hacks and tips – and cure it all the way!

Martin Meyer

Legal & Disclaimer

Legal & Disclaimer

The information contained in this book is not designed to replace or take the place of any form of medicine or professional medical advice. The information in this book has been provided for educational and entertainment purposes only.

The information contained in this book has been compiled from sources deemed reliable, and it is accurate to the best of the Author's knowledge; however, the Author cannot guarantee its accuracy and validity and cannot be held liable for any errors or omissions. Changes are periodically made to this book. You must consult your doctor or get professional medical advice before using any of the suggested remedies, techniques, or information in this book.

Upon using the information contained in this book, you agree to hold harmless the Author from and against any damages, costs, and expenses, including any legal fees potentially resulting from the application of any of the information provided by this guide. This disclaimer applies to any damages or injury caused by the use and application, whether directly or indirectly, of any advice or information presented, whether for breach of contract, tort, negligence, personal injury, criminal intent, or under any other cause of action.

You agree to accept all risks of using the information presented inside this book. You need to consult a professional medical practitioner in order to ensure you are both able and healthy enough to participate in this program.

Table of Contents

Introduction

Diabetes mellitus is described as abnormally high amounts of glucose in the blood which can occur due to many reasons, such as inheritance, malfunctioning of pancreas or complete absence of insulin producing cells.

At the point when the measure of glucose in the blood increases, e.g., after a feast, it triggers the arrival of the hormone insulin from the pancreas. Insulin animates muscles and fat cells to expel glucose from the blood and invigorates the liver to metabolize glucose, creating the glucose level to reduce to typical levels.

Blood glucose level is a vital measure of your wellbeing. In case you're attempting to deal with your blood glucose levels, this eBook can offer assistance! With the most recent instruments and systems, you can make strides today to screen your condition, avoid genuine intricacies and feel better while living with diabetes.

Anyway, would you say you are diabetic or are at danger for diabetes? Do you stress over your glucose? At that point, you've come to the ideal spot. The accompanying eBook contains the accurate data which will help you control your blood glucose level and manage it nicely to the point where you can cure your condition and bid farewell to the ever-haunting complications of this disease.

Section A: Overview

The number of individuals with diabetes is expanding alarmingly fast and is approaching 500 million per annum. This is a world pandemic. Will somebody in your family be influenced next? Your mom, cousin, father, your tyke? Or maybe you? Is your blood as of now too sweet?

Those influenced by the most widely recognized type of diabetes (type 2) typically never recover their wellbeing. Rather, we underestimate that they'll turn into somewhat more broken down for consistently that passes by. With time, they require more medications. Yet, at some point or another intricacies develop. Visual deficiency. Dialysis because of flawed kidneys. Dementia or perhaps, death.

What is Diabetes?

Diabetes is a condition where the measure of glucose in your blood is too high in light of the fact that the body can't utilize it legitimately.

This is on the grounds that your pancreas doesn't deliver any insulin or insufficient insulin, to offer glucose some assistance with entering your body's cells – or the insulin that is created does not work appropriately.

Types

In individuals with diabetes, glucose levels stay high. This might be on the grounds that insulin is not being delivered by any stretch of the imagination, is not made at adequate levels, or is not as successful as it ought to be. The most widely recognized types of diabetes are:

- Type 1 diabetes (5%), which is an immune system issue, and
- Type 2 diabetes (95%), which is connected with heftiness.

Gestational diabetes is a type of diabetes that happens during pregnancy, and different types of diabetes are exceptionally uncommon and are created by a solitary mutation or transformation.

Origin

Type 2 diabetes is by a long shot, the most widely recognized structure (around 90% of all cases) and the one which is expanding the most. It fundamentally influences overweight individuals in middle age or later. It isn't extraordinary that the influenced individual likewise has hypertension and terrible cholesterol levels.

In short, in diabetes, the body has an undeniably harder time to handle all the sugar in the blood. A lot of the glucose bringing down hormone-insulin is created, yet, it's insufficient as insulin affectability diminishes. At the moment of analysis, type 2 diabetics typically have ten times more insulin in their bodies than ordinary people. As a symptom, this insulin stores fat and causes weight pick up, something that has regularly been in advancement for a long time before the malady was analyzed.

Risk factors

Being overweight, physically latent and eating the wrong foods all add to our danger of creating type 2 diabetes.

Point to ponder!

Drinking only one bottle of pop every day can raise our danger of developing type 2 diabetes by 22%.

The researchers trust that the effect of sugary sodas on diabetes danger might be an immediate one, as opposed to just an impact on body weight.

The danger of creating type 2 diabetes is additionally more noteworthy as we get more established. Specialists are not totally beyond any doubt why, but rather say that as we age we tend to put on weight and turn out to be less physically dynamic.

Those with a nearby relative who had/has type 2 diabetes, especially the individuals of Middle Eastern, African, or South

Asian region, likewise have a higher danger of building up the illness.

Men whose testosterone levels are low have been found to have a higher danger of creating type 2 diabetes too.

Sign and symptoms

This diseases can cause a wide range of signs and symptoms, including:

- Thirst
- Fatigue
- Excessive urination
- Hunger
- Dry mouth

- Blurry vision
- Weight loss
- Wounds that won't heal
- Cloudy thinking
- Irritability

A look on pre-diabetes

By far, most of the patients with type 2 diabetes, at first, had prediabetes. Their blood glucose levels were higher than ordinary, yet not sufficiently high to justify a diabetes conclusion. Technically, the cells in the body are getting to be impervious to insulin.

Researchers have demonstrated that even at the prediabetes stage, some harm to the circulatory framework and the heart starts to pursue.

Prediabetes is a reminder that you're on the way to diabetes. Be that as it may, it's not very late to turn things around. On the off chance that you have it, your blood sugar level is higher than it ought to be, however not in the diabetes range. Individuals used to call it "marginal" diabetes too, therefore.

Symptoms and other diseases

Typically, your body makes a hormone called insulin to control your glucose. You won't have the capacity to make enough insulin in the wake of eating, or your body won't react to insulin legitimately. Prediabetes makes you more prone to get coronary illness or have a stroke. Yet, the good news is, you can make a move to lower those dangers.

Diagnosis and Analysis

Your specialist will give you one of three basic blood tests:

Hemoglobin A1C (or normal glucose) test.

This blood test demonstrates your normal glucose level for as long as 3 to 4 months. Specialists can utilize it to analyze prediabetes or diabetes or, on the off chance that you definitely know you have diabetes, it demonstrates whether it's under control. The outcomes are:

- Diabetes: 6.5% or above
- Prediabetes: 5.7 to 6.4%
- Ordinary: 5.6% or less

You might need to take the test again to affirm the outcomes.

Fasting plasma glucose test.

You won't be allowed to eat for 8 hours before taking this blood test. The outcomes are:

- Diabetes if your glucose is 126 or higher
- Prediabetes if your glucose is 100-125
- Perfectly normal if your glucose is under 100

Oral glucose resistance test.

To begin with, you'll take the fasting glucose test. After this, you'll be asked to drink a sugary arrangement. Two hours after that, you'll take another blood test. The outcomes are:

- Diabetes if your glucose is 200 or higher after the second test
- Prediabetes if your glucose is 140-199 after the second test
- Considerable if your glucose is under 140 after the second test

Empirical management

A great number of people with type 2 diabetes don't take insulin. You might be considering how you can accomplish tight control without it.

One route is to shed pounds. Shedding abundance pounds might convey your glucose levels down to ordinary. The way to getting more fit and keeping it off is changing your conduct with the goal that you eat less and practice more. Your specialist ought to work with you to discover an eating and practice arrangement you can stick to.

Other risks for diabetics

- As the danger of cardiovascular infection is much higher for a diabetic, it is pivotal that circulatory strain and cholesterol levels are observed consistently.
- As smoking may seriously affect cardiovascular wellbeing, diabetics ought to quit smoking.
- Hypoglycemia - low blood glucose - can badly affect the patient. Hyperglycemia - when blood glucose is too high - can likewise badly affect the patient.

Regardless of the possibility that you don't have to get in shape, activity is useful in controlling your blood glucose levels. It makes your cells take glucose out of the blood.

You should check your blood glucose frequently. You ought to choose with your specialist how frequently. Once per day or even once every week might be sufficient for a few individuals with type 2 diabetes.

In the event that practice and great dietary patterns are insufficient to hold your glucose under control, you specialist might recommend pills. Furthermore, if these don't work, you might need to take intramuscular insulin. Individuals with type 2 diabetes should converse with their specialists before beginning tight control under a suitable plan.

Section B: Dietary management

The issue for diabetics is that the body experiences issues holding glucose levels down. The blood turns too sweet. So where does sugar in the blood originate from?

Sugar in the blood originates from the nourishment that we eat. The sustenance's that transform into various sorts of sugar when they achieve the stomach are called starches. This implies sugar (as in pop, natural product squeeze, treat) and starches (as in bread, pasta, rice and potatoes).

The starch, in for instance bread, is separated to glucose in the stomach. At the point when glucose enters the circulation system, it's called glucose.

The more starches we eat in a supper, the more sugar is consumed into the circulation system. The more sugar that is consumed by the circulation system, the higher the glucose will be.

Diabetes, an evil.

- Individuals with diabetes are twice as liable to create coronary illness as somebody without diabetes.
- Bariatric surgery can lessen the side effects of diabetes in fat individuals.
- Great control of diabetes altogether decreases the danger of creating complexities and keeps intricacies from deteriorating.
- Diabetes costs $174 billion every year, incorporating $116 billion in direct restorative costs.

An enlisted dietitian can help you set up together an eating routine taking into account your wellbeing objectives, tastes and way of life and can give profitable data on the best way to change your dietary patterns.

Foods to eat

Make the most of your calories with these nutritious nourishments:

Fiber-rich nourishments

Dietary fiber incorporates all parts of plant nourishments that your body can't process or assimilate. Fiber can diminish the danger of coronary illness and control glucose levels. Nourishments high in fiber incorporate fruits, nuts, organic products, vegetables (beans, peas and lentils), and wheat grain and wheat flour.

Sound starches

Amid absorption, sugars and starches separate into blood glucose. Concentrate on the most beneficial sugars, for example, vegetables, natural products, vegetables (peas, lentils and beans), entire grains and low-fat dairy items.

Heart friendly fish

Eat heart-solid fish at any rate twice every week. Fish can be a decent distinct option for high-fat meats. For instance, cod and halibut have less aggregate fat, soaked fat, and cholesterol than do meat and poultry. Fish, for example, mackerel, salmon, sardines, and bluefish are rich in omega-3 i.e. unsaturated fats, which advances heart wellbeing by bringing down blood fats called TAGs. Be that as it may, maintain a strategic distance from browned fish with abnormal amounts of mercury, for example, swordfish, ruler mackerel, and tilefish.

Cholesterol

Wellsprings of cholesterol incorporate high-fat dairy items and high-fat creature proteins, shellfish, egg yolks, liver, and other organ meats. Go for close to 300 milligrams (mg) of cholesterol a day.

Good fats

Nourishments containing polyunsaturated and monounsaturated fats, for example, avocados, pecans, almonds, walnuts, and canola, olive and nut oils can bring down your cholesterol levels. Eat them sparingly, in any case, as all fats are high in calories. High-fat dairy items and creature proteins, for example, hamburger, franks, wiener and bacon contain soaked fats. Get close to 7 percent of your day by day calories from immersed fat.

There are a couple of various ways to deal with making diabetes eating routine that keeps your blood glucose level inside of an ordinary reach. With a dietitian's help, you might discover one or a blend of strategies that works for you.

Proved diet to reverse Diabetes in a month!

This is the most important part of this book! If you follow this diet bellow I will guarantee that you'll reverse your diabetes within two months(most likely 1 month). This is a proven diet by scientific studies that haven't been released to the public. You'll have to stick to this diet and consume nothing else!

The diet emphasizes consumption of greens and other non-starchy vegetables, such as onions, mushrooms, eggplant, peppers, tomatoes and cauliflower, in unlimited quantity. High glycimic, high carbohydrate foods are reduced, while beans, peas, squash and intact gains are permitted. Nuts and seeds are the primary source of fat, while animal products are limited to 10 percent of calories or less.

1) At least one large green salad a day, with inclusion of a nut/seed derived salad dressing.

2) One bowl of vegetable-bean soup daily.

3) 1 - 2 ounces of raw seeds and nuts daily (usually in salad dressing recipe)

4) Approximately 3-4 fresh fruits a day.

5) One large serving of steamed or stewed greens, with mushrooms, onions and other low-starch veggies.

6) Only one serving a day of non-bean starch, such as squash, steel cut oats, brown/wild rice.

7) Exclusion of white flour, sweets and oils, while limiting animal products to 12 ounces per week.

Foods to avoid

To maintain a healthy routine you should avoid the below mentioned food products and keep a safe distance from all of them.

Sugary Foods

Pop, desserts, pastries, and different food that are made basically of sugar are viewed as low-quality starches. Not just are these nourishments ailing in dietary worth, they can likewise bring about a sharp spike in your glucose and lead to weight issues, both of which worsen diabetes complexities.

Rather than fulfilling your sweet tooth with treats, confection, cake, or pop, go after delectable organic products, for example, apples, berries, pears, or oranges. These superb starches contain a lot of fiber to back off the ingestion of glucose, so they're a far superior decision for glucose control.

Fruit Juices

While fiber-rich entire organic products are viewed as solid starches for individuals with diabetes, natural product juice is another story. Individuals with diabetes ought to abstain from drinking juice, even 100 percent natural product juice. Natural product juice contains more nourishment than pop and other sugary beverages, however, the issue is that squeezes have concentrated measures of organic product sugar and in this manner cause your glucose to shoot up. Additionally, tasting organic product juice doesn't top you off the same way that eating a bit of natural product does. In the event that you need an invigorating beverage, go for zero-calorie plain or normally seasoned seltzer with a spritz of lemon or lime.

Dried Fruits

Albeit dried organic product contains fiber and numerous supplements, the parchedness process cause natural products' characteristic sugars to get super-focused. While eating on raisins or dried apricots is preferable for you over eating a treat, despite everything it'll send your glucose taking off. Avoid the dried leafy foods stay with new organic product alternatives, for example, grapefruit, melon, strawberries, and peaches.

Bundled Snacks and Baked Goods

Beside all the sugar, junky white flour, and additives they contain, bundled snacks and prepared merchandise like chips, pretzels, saltines, treats, donuts, and nibble cakes frequently have trans fats. Trans fats expand your bad cholesterol, bring down your good cholesterol, and raise your danger of coronary illness.

Furthermore, they are significantly a greater number of hazardous than soaked fats for individuals who have sort 2 diabetes. Truth be told, no measure of trans fats is considered safe for you to join in your eating routine. The uplifting news is that trans fats are currently recorded directly after the measure of immersed fats on sustenance marks, making it less demanding to keep away from them.

Using food/drinks as medicine

Much sooner than specialists and drug was normally utilized, savvy tribal older folks would search out mending herbs and plants for their group and nourishment that could be connected prescriptively to cure medical conditions. Gradually during that time, man has moved far from the mending force of nature and towards endorsing bundled engineered drugs and manufactured solutions for managing sickness.

Here are some tried-and-tested foods that are meant to lower your blood sugar and control your diabetes – all by the ultimate power of nature!

- **Turmeric:** Research in the previous decade has demonstrated that turmeric helps against diabetes as well as washes down the liver, offers characteristic calming properties, secures against bosom and prostate tumors, and moderates the development of Alzheimer's and type 2 diabetes. Curcumin is the key substance in turmeric which scientists identify as the wellspring of its large number of mending forces.
- **Fenugreek:** Another substance used to zest Indian food, fenugreek, additionally offers assurance against diabetes. Fenugreek has the additional advantage of boosting male sex drive, upgrading liver capacity, and bringing down cholesterol. It also keeps the sugar levels in control thus helping diabetics a lot.
- **Brown chocolate:** Analysts in a study recommend that with some restraint, dim chocolate made with negligible preparing

are a more beneficial type of intermittent liberality than most different desserts, yet their calorie content still makes them a potential risk.

- **Cocoa powder:** Cocoa powder and heating chocolate contain the largest amounts of the flavonoids in charge of the positive wellbeing impacts connected with chocolate. Dull chocolate gives less of these flavonoids while white chocolate has none.
- **Beans:** Beans can direct blood glucose and insulin levels to a low level. They can avoid diabetes, or minimize its risk in some individuals. They likewise bring down cholesterol levels and offer against oxidant properties. Red beans offer the most astounding results against oxidant levels, trailed by dark beans.

While medications are vital in life undermining circumstances, if long haul conditions can be made do with eating regimen and life changes, then utilizing sustenance as prescription must be considered as a wonderful method for handling the issue and forestalling future wellbeing issues.

Section C: Alternative approach

At the point when a person has diabetes, keeping up tight glucose control is one part of ailment administration that, however, does not paint the whole picture. Notwithstanding medicines, for example, insulin infusions, patients might utilize corresponding and elective treatments to better deal with their diabetes. These treatments might mean to regard the brain and also the body.

Before you start such medicines, it is vital to perceive that there is restricted confirmation on how well they do or don't function. Additionally, in light of the fact that supplements are "all-normal" does not mean they won't meddle with diabetes prescriptions or different medicines. Individuals with diabetes ought to dependably enlighten their doctor concerning any option treatments they are taking to guarantee security.

Minimizing stress

Anxiety is a physical and mental response to saw peril. Conditions that seen wild or require enthusiastic and behavioral change have a tendency to be seen as a danger.

At the point when the body and psyche sense a risk, they get prepared to either run or battle. Whether the risk is genuine or envisioned, the body gets ready for survival by turning up some real capacities while turning others down. In either case, after all these progressions are not kidding and after some time are unsafe.

27

Effects of stress

With mental anxiety, the body pumps out hormones without much of any result. Neither battling nor escaping is any assistance when the "adversary" is your own brain.

In individuals with diabetes, anxiety can modify blood glucose levels in two ways:

- Individuals under anxiety may not take great consideration of themselves. They might drink more liquor or practice less. They might overlook, or not have time, to check their glucose levels or plan great dinners.
- Stress hormones might likewise adjust blood glucose levels specifically.

Tips to sooth stress:

1. Dodge liquor, caffeine, and worthless worries around evening time.
2. Keep up a somewhat cool temperature in your rest surroundings.
3. Obstruct out all light and disturbing noises.
4. Go to bed early to consistently build up a rest plan.

Keeping weight under control

Keep up (or come back to) a sound weight. Weight is one of the main danger variables for creating type 2 diabetes. It might console to realize that if you are overweight, dropping a moderate 5 percent to 10 percent of your weight cuts your danger of creating diabetes down the middle. A low-calorie, low-fat eating regimen is prescribed as the most ideal approach to control your weight and avert diabetes.

Fruits and vegetables

Concentrate on natural products. Eating an assortment of leafy foods consistently might cut your diabetes hazard by as much as 22 percent, as indicated by results from a 12-year dietary investigation of 21,831 grown-ups. Your danger lessening is straightforwardly identified with what number of products of the soil you expend.

High calorie drinks

Remove the sugary beverages from your diet. Wellbeing information from 43,960 dark ladies demonstrated that ladies who drink two or more sweet beverages a day have a 25 to 30 percent higher danger of diabetes than their associates.

Starting to exercise

Get moving. Getting no less than 30 minutes of exercise a day can offer you some assistance with achieving your weight reduction objectives and cut your diabetes hazard however exercise likewise beneficially affects glucose and insulin levels. Decreased TV time can also help. The hours you spend sitting in front of the TV are connected with diabetes hazard.

Exercise

When you have type 2 diabetes, physical action is a critical part of your treatment. It's likewise vital to have a solid supper arrangement and keep up your blood glucose level through prescriptions or insulin, if fundamental.

How it helps

In the event that you stay fit and dynamic for the duration of your life, you'll have the capacity to better control your diabetes and keep your blood glucose level in the right range. Controlling your blood glucose level is crucial to anticipating long haul complexities, for example, nerve damage, retinopathies and kidney diseases.

Exercise has such a large number of advantages, however, the greatest one is that it makes it less demanding to control your glucose level. Individuals with type 2 diabetes have an excess of glucose in their blood, either in light of the fact that their body doesn't sufficiently deliver insulin to process it or in light of the fact that their body doesn't utilize insulin appropriately.

Before you begin exercising...

At the point when the vast majority are determined to have type 2 diabetes, they are overweight, so the thought of practicing is especially overwhelming. For your wellbeing, you need to begin on a decent, sensible exercise arrangement, however, to start with, you should talk with your specialist.

Regular exercise

In either case, exercise can lessen the glucose in your blood.
Muscles can utilize glucose without insulin when you're
working out. At the end of the day, it doesn't make a difference
in case you're insulin safe or on the off chance that you don't
have enough insulin: when you exercise, your muscles get the
glucose they require, and thus, your blood glucose level goes
down.

Exercise can likewise help individuals with type 2 diabetes
maintain a strategic distance from long term consequences,
particularly heart issues. Individuals with diabetes are
powerless to creating blocked blood vessels (arteriosclerosis),
which can prompt a heart attack. Exercise keeps your heart
much healthier. Besides, exercise offers you some assistance
with maintaining great cholesterol—and that offers you great
help with avoiding arteriosclerosis.

Essential oils

These oils are nature's powerful essence and contain a wide range of concoction fixings that are extricated from plants through refining, a procedure of sanitizing fluids by bubbling and gathering its vapors.

- **Coriander:** Cilantro or coriander started from western Asia and eastern Mediterranean district. Customarily, coriander has been utilized as a mix to cure digestive issues like looseness of the bowels in kids, colic agony, flatulence and anorexia. For diabetes, Coriander advances low blood glucose levels by increasing the insulin emission in the pancreas. What's more, this oil is additionally known to produce insulin at the cell level.
- **Cinnamon:** Expending Cinnamon orally might facilitate the indications of diabetes. Research has demonstrated that Cinnamon can diminish the levels of glucose, triglycerides and cholesterol in the body. Other than that, this oil can battle disease, diminish aggravation and parity glucose levels. It has regular antifungal and antiviral properties to battle contamination and alongside that, it is a characteristic insusceptible promoter.
- **Fenugreek Oil:** One of the studies directed on greasy rats found that fenugreek could fundamentally increase the insulin levels affectability in the body. With further research, it was reasoned that Fenugreek focuses on the manifestations of the infection as well as makes the life of a diabetic less keeping so as to demand him crisp and invigorated for the duration of the day.

- **Citrus Oils blend:** Diabetes is an ailment that influences pancreas as well as numerous organs and procedures all through the body including the vision. Mixes of Citrus oils can bolster the visual framework and the significant organs, for example, the liver as they are rich in regular cell reinforcements.
- **Black Pepper Oil:** Dark Pepper can control and even counteract hypertension and type II diabetes.

Black pepper!

A study held in 2013 states that the oil of black pepper normally controls two catalysts that separate starch into glucose. This impact standardizes glucose levels and backs off the assimilation of glucose.

Herbs and supplements

Herbs and supplements are probably the most famous CAM treatments for individuals with diabetes. The U.S. Sustenance and Drug Administration does not consider these treatments "prescriptions." Therefore, they are not managed.

The following are probably the most famous supplements utilized with diabetes.

Alpha-Lipoic Acid

Alpha-lipoic corrosive is a cancer prevention agent discovered actually in nourishments such as spinach, broccoli, and potatoes. The supplement is thought to lessen nerve harm identified with diabetes (diabetic neuropathy) and enhance the body's capacity to utilize insulin. A few studies bolster the utilization of this supplement for neuropathy.

Aloe Vera

You can apply gel from this regular family unit plant topically or take it as an oral supplement. The gel is generally used to mitigate blazes. Two clinical trials found that aloe vera taken orally brought down the fasting glucose amid a six-week trial period. In any case, the studies did not cover long term use.

Cinnamon

Studies on this well-known diabetes supplement have given extremely conflicting results. By Mayo Clinic, a few studies demonstrate that cinnamon can upgrade insulin affectability while others have found no impacts. In the event that cinnamon is useful, its advantages are negligible.

Chromium

Patients with diabetes have been appeared to lose more chromium in their pee. This is thought to influence insulin resistance. A United States study that deliberates the adequacy of chromium supplements crosswise over 180 patients discovered patients who took 500 µg of the supplement twice per day saw enhanced HbA1C levels than those in the fake treatment bunch. Be that as it may, different studies don't bolster these discoveries.

Garlic

Garlic, is a prominent supplement, yet examine on its belongings in individuals with diabetes is insignificant. Clinical trials in patients with type 2 diabetes who took garlic did not demonstrate changes in glucose or insulin levels. Some clinical trials discovered garlic brought down aggregate cholesterol levels and circulatory strain levels.

Section D: Curing Diabetes

Fighting food addiction

Wouldn't you love it if our body size and blood sugars remain the same even if we eat anything we want?

One noteworthy reason this doesn't happen needs to do with our weight control plans. When you devour starch and refined sugar, these nourishments enter the circulation system rapidly, bringing on a sugar spike. Your body then creates the hormone insulin to drive that sugar from your circulation system into cells. Yet, after some time, unreasonable levels of insulin can make your muscle cells lose affectability to the hormone, prompting type 2 diabetes and coronary illness. Your fat cells are another story: They generally stay touchy. Insulin spikes lock fat into them, so you can't utilize it for vitality.

Begin your feast with Salad

It douses up starch and sugar. Solvent fiber from the mash of plants, for example, beans, apples, carrots, and oranges swells like a wipe in your guts and traps starch and sugar in the specialties between its particles. A decent approach to guarantee that you get enough dissolvable fiber is to have a plate of mixed greens—ideally some time recently, as opposed to after, you eat a starch.

Include a dash of vinegar in your daily meals

It moderates the breakdown of starch into sugar. The high acidic corrosive substance in vinegar deactivates amylase, the catalyst that transforms starch into sugar. You ought to devour vinegar toward the beginning of your feast. Placed it in serving of mixed greens dressing or sprinkle two or three tablespoons of meat or vegetables. Vinegar draws out the kind of sustenance, as salt does.

Keeping sugar level in check

Blood (glucose) monitoring is the fundamental device you need to check your diabetes control. This check lets you know your blood glucose level at any one time.

When you complete the blood glucose check, record your outcomes and audit them to perceive how nutrition, movement, and anxiety influence your blood glucose. Examine your blood glucose record to check whether your level is too high or too low a few days in succession at about the same time. On the off chance that the same thing continues happening, it may be a great opportunity to change your arrangement. Work with your specialist or diabetes instructor to realize what your outcomes mean for you. This requires significant investment. Ask your specialist or medical attendant if you ought to report results out of a specific reach without a moment's delay by telephone.

Remember that blood glucose comes about frequently trigger solid emotions. Blood glucose numbers can leave you steamed, befuddled, baffled, irate, or down. It's anything but difficult to utilize the numbers to judge yourself. Advise yourself that your blood glucose level is an approach to track how well your diabetes care arrangement is working. It is not a judgment of you as a man. The outcomes might demonstrate to you require an adjustment in your diabetes arrangement.

TAKE- AWAY MESSAGE! Use the provided alternative management options, take help from herbs and dietary modification, team up with your doctor and device a plan to keep your blood sugar spike at bay. With trial and error, there will come a time when you won't have to stress the need to take insulin shots and checking your sugar levels because your diabetes will be largely controlled – and hopefully cured!

Conclusion

Diabetes is a genuine illness that retards our quality of life if not kept under control. Patients with diabetes can be taught how to control their diabetes by controlling what they eat, checking their glucose a few times each day, and working out.

If not controlled, diabetes can prompt genuine complications, for example, kidney diseases, visual impairment, and even death. It is less demanding to forestall diabetes than to treat it.

Diabetes is a moderate killer with no known reparable medicines. In any case, its symptoms can be decreased through legitimate mindfulness and promising treatment. Three noteworthy inconveniences are identified with visual deficiency, kidney harm, and heart attack. It is imperative to keep the blood glucose levels of patients under strict control for maintaining a strategic distance from the inconveniences.

One of the challenges with tight control of glucose levels in the blood is that such endeavors might prompt hypoglycemia that makes many serious difficulties than an increased level of blood glucose, leading to lactoacidosis, coma and ultimate death. Specialists now search for more solid options for diabetes treatment. The objective of this eBook is to give a general thought of the momentum status of diabetes examination and how to control diabetes in proper and regulated manner. Use the provided information, tips and management strategies to counter the disease progression, improve your disease prognosis and lead a healthy, diabetes-free life.
Good luck.
Martin Meyer

www.ingramcontent.com/pod-product-compliance
Lightning Source LLC
Chambersburg PA
CBHW071308280526
45788CB00004B/1858